Help! I Have Head Lice

Everything You Want to Know About Head Lice and How to Get Rid of It

2019
***ISBN:** 9781696968133*

By

Shannon Hartup, *The Lice Lady*

*To all those who suffer with head lice,
this book is dedicated to you.*

Table of Contents

Table of Contents continued

Introduction

Hi. I'm Shannon, a professional head lice technician. I've written this book to give the everyday person the know-how to get rid of headlice and to protect themselves and their loved ones from being infested with head lice.

 Follow the simple, illustrated step-by-step instructions in these pages and you will successfully eradicate head lice from your home or office, children, clients, students, patients and yourself, using products you already own.

I share the method I've used on myself and my clients. It works, and anyone can do this using no chemicals or expensive merchandise.

Be assured, *all* your questions about head lice are covered in this book and on my website:

www.helpihaveheadlice.com.

Learn how to get lice free and stay lice free, for every hair type.

At the end of the book, you will find the children's story *Help! I Have Head Lice*, written by Bev Gipson. I hope you and your children enjoy it!

PART I:
Instructions
on
Head Lice

Chapter One

What Are Head Lice and What Do They Look Like?

Head lice are parasitic bugs that live exclusively on our heads. Your beard and any other part of your body that has hair (such as arm pits, legs, privates, eyebrows, etc.) is not at risk for head lice. If you are bald, you are not at risk of having or ever getting head lice.

Why? Head lice claws are formed to scale human hair only. When they are not on a scalp with hair, they move awkwardly and slowly. If they can't return to a scalp with hair, they will die. Our heads provide everything they need to survive - warmth, food (blood), moisture, and a place to mate and lay their eggs.

A single head lice is called a "louse".

The life cycle of a head louse has three stages: NITS, NYMPH, and ADULT.

NITS are head lice eggs. They are often confused for dandruff or hair spray residue. Consequently, they are hard to detect. Nits are laid by the adult female and are found at the nape of the hair shaft nearest the scalp. The first egg is usually laid one-fourth inch/0.5 cm from the scalp. If head lice go untreated and thrive, nits may be laid one on top of another.

Nits are attached to the hair with a glue-like substance that keeps them cemented to the hair. They are usually yellow to white, but I've come across darker eggs in my practice.

Nits take six to ten days to hatch.

NYMPHS are the second stage. The nymph looks like an adult head louse but is about the size of a pinhead. It takes one week for the nymph to become an adult.

ADULTS are the final stage. An adult louse is about the size of a sesame seed: 0.08 to

0.12 inches. They are white/gray in color but once they fill up with blood, they turn brown to black. Like mosquitos, head lice feed on our blood. Human blood provides all the sustenance head lice need.

More females than males are hatched. Females are usually larger than males. Females mate only once with a male and then they lay up to eight nits per day. A female will lay 150 to 240 eggs in her adult life.

Adult lice can live up to 30 days on a person's head.

Head lice feed on blood several times a day and depend on our warmth, moisture and blood to survive. Without blood meals and moisture, the louse will die within one to two days. They cannot live beyond 48 hours off a host.

Each bug has six legs with claws that move extremely fast up and down human hair. Head lice do not have knees or wings. They trapeze from hair strand to hair strand with their tiny claws.

As unpleasant as it is, lice leave behind unwanted residue from living on us. We were, after all, their home. Egg shells, exoskeleton, and their droppings sometimes show up after they're cleared from our hair. Don't be alarmed. These will all be washed or brushed out of our hair in time. If you have a lice comb, you can comb them out.

The two pictures below are of an adult headlice. The bottom one is an adult head lice on a Q-Tip. Head lice are transparent, like a shrimp, until they eat, then they appear brown to dark brown.

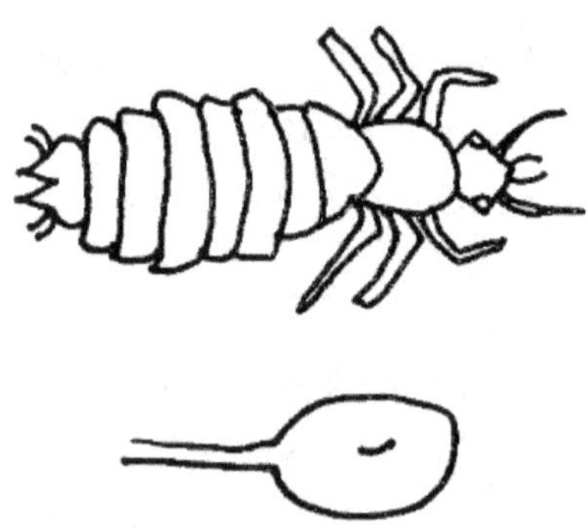

***

Chapter Two

Where Do Head Lice Come From? and Other Questions.

On my website *www.helpihaveheadlice.com* I have a page called *Head Lice Facts* where I have a wealth of information about head lice and have posted the itchiest questions about these pesky creatures. Below are some of the most frequently asked questions.

1. *Can head lice infest a home, like bed bugs?*

Head lice need a warm, moist environment to thrive and must feed every 3-4 hours. When head lice are not on a human host, they will either dry up or starve to death within 24 hours. A very hearty head louse may live 48 hours once off of a host. You can conceivably lock up your home for 48 hours, and upon returning, every bug will be dead.

2. *Can our pets get head lice from us?*

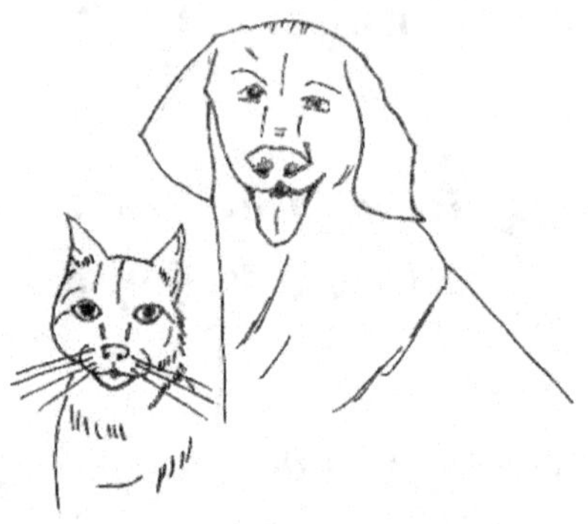

Fortunately, our pets cannot carry or contract head lice. Head lice are human parasites and can only survive on our scalp and on our blood.

3. *Does everyone's scalp itch when they get head lice?*

Itching is caused by our reaction to the louse's saliva. It is also caused by the movement of the bugs when they scurry around our scalp. Not everyone reacts to head lice saliva or their movements the same way. Some people do not itch at all and some have chronic itching due to the bites and the movement of the bugs.

4. *How do people get head lice?*

95% of head lice are spread through head to head contact, but they can also be transmitted through hair accessories, clothing, hats, pillowcases, and other items.

5. *Do head lice drown?*

Head lice can live in water for up to 8 hours.

6. *If a head lice egg falls off of a human head, can it still hatch?*

Yes. However, circumstances for an egg to hatch successfully have to be near perfect: a warm, moist place to incubate, and then a host to feed upon *immediately* after hatching.

7. *What percentage of USA schools will experience a head lice outbreak in a single year?*

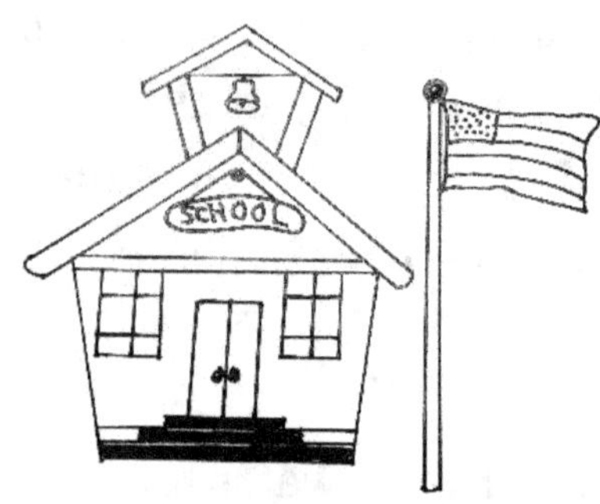

80% of schools will experience a head lice outbreak.

8. *Do head lice carry diseases?*

Head Lice do not transmit or carry diseases. The only medical issue that becomes a concern is infection due to the host scratching their bites.

9. *Is it true only people with dirty hair get head lice?*

No. Head lice prefer clean hair but will live in dirty hair.

10. *Where does the word 'lousy' come from?*

You guessed it! The word "lousy" is derived from "louse" as in, "It sure is lousy to get head lice!" And the phrase "nit pickin'" as in, "You nit pickin' louse!" is in reference to picking nits (lice eggs) out of someone's hair.

***

Chapter Three

What Are Super Lice?

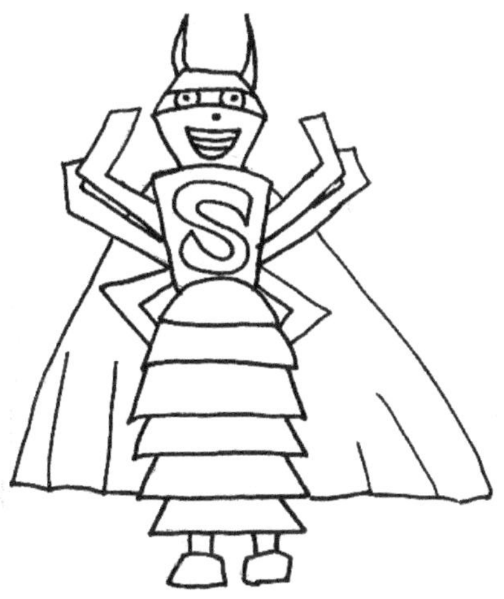

Head lice have slowly become immune to common treatments due to overexposure to insecticides over the past 20-30 years. Consequently, this bred resistance in the parasites and created a 'super lice.'

"Super lice" now make up 97% of head lice cases. The bugs have not changed in appearance, just in resilience to the most popular treatments.

But there are still safe and successful ways to get rid of these pests.

Keep reading. It can be simpler than you think to get rid of head lice.

***

Chapter Four

Do I Need a Lice Comb?

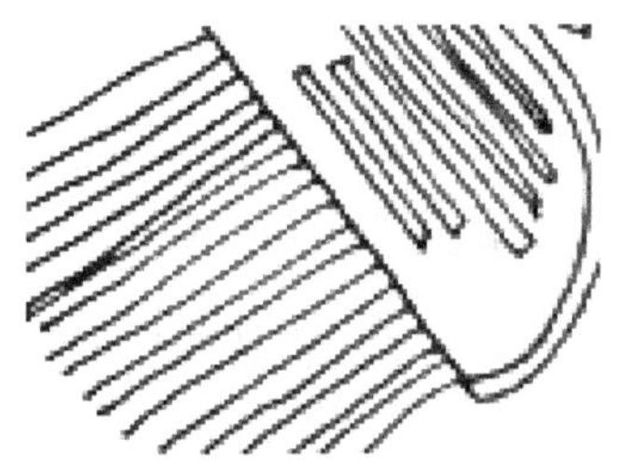

Unless you have a severe case of headlice, you probably don't need a head lice comb. However, a licc comb will remove the residue, nit shells and dead lice bugs following a treatment. These will be brushed or washed out of your hair eventually without using a lice comb.

There is only one kind of comb that I use and suggest to my clients to own. It's called *Nit Free Terminator Comb*. It has stainless steel tines that pull the eggs out. The comb is well made and should last for years.

Many schools insist their students be cleared of all bugs and nits before returning to school. If this is the case, you will need a head lice comb to pull the eggs and residue out.

If eggs are visible in your hair and this bothers you, it's probably a good idea to get the comb.

Eggs are easy to spot because they are usually white and look like dandruff, but they don't flake off like dandruff. I have found brown and black eggs on clients, but most often the eggs are white.

Eggs are attached to hair with a substance the consistency of glue that the female secretes to attach the egg to our hair. Consequently, they must be pulled off of our hair strands by a good comb or your fingernails.

However, you can get rid of head lice without using a comb. I explain how in the following chapters.

I'm often asked how to clean a lice comb. It's simple. After you have used your comb place it in your freezer for 12-24 hours and that will kill any eggs or bugs that may be stuck to the tines. After you remove it from the freezer, wash it in hot, soapy water, and use a toothbrush to brush the tines clean.

I do not recommend boiling the combs as several of mine have rusted. With proper care your comb should last for years.

***

Chapter Five

Kinky Hair, Coily Hair and Natural Hair

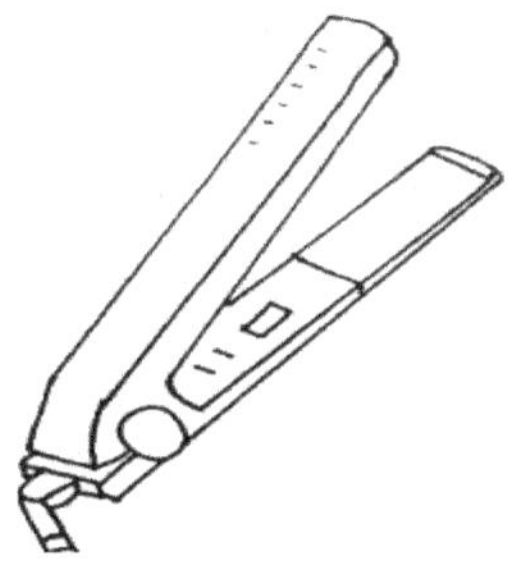

Kinky hair, coily hair and natural hair are more difficult to treat because it is extremely difficult to remove the eggs and bugs with a head lice comb. If you have a very mild case of head lice and don't mind the presence of eggs in your hair, you can skip using a lice comb altogether. In the next chapters this procedure is explained: you will just apply the oil or Dimethicone that I recommend in

Chapter Six, using a liberal amount to cover every strand of hair and your entire scalp. Skip Chapter Seven, and instead follow the instructions in Chapter Eight (which is Step Three). You will be treating yourself only three times: *Day One, Day Five* and *Day Eleven*. By Day Eleven you will be completely head lice free.

To know which days, you will need to treat yourself, begin by counting five days after your first treatment. For example, if your first treatment is March 2, Day Five is March 7 and Day Eleven is March 13.

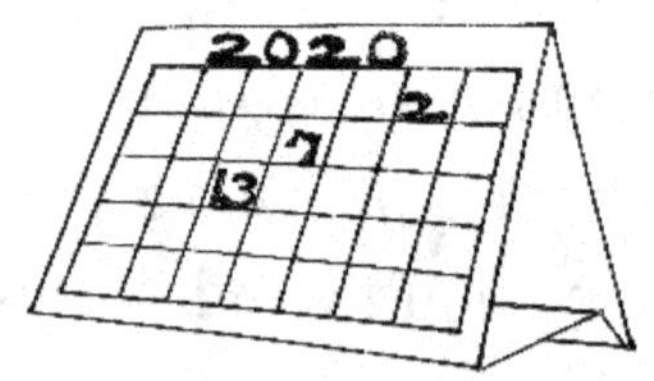

If you have a serious case of head lice and/or need to remove all signs of eggs and their residue, then simply using the oil won't work.

You will need to straighten your hair in order to do a comb-out. If you are unfamiliar with the procedure on how to straighten your hair, there are many good YouTube videos that give step by step instructions and are easy to follow.

That being said, you will need a good hair straightener. Because kinky, coily and natural hair can be more sensitive to heat and thus harder to straighten, use a heat protectant on your hair and extra conditioning. Once the hair is straightened, follow the steps about combing outlined in Chapters Seven and Eight.

***

Chapter Six

How To Start

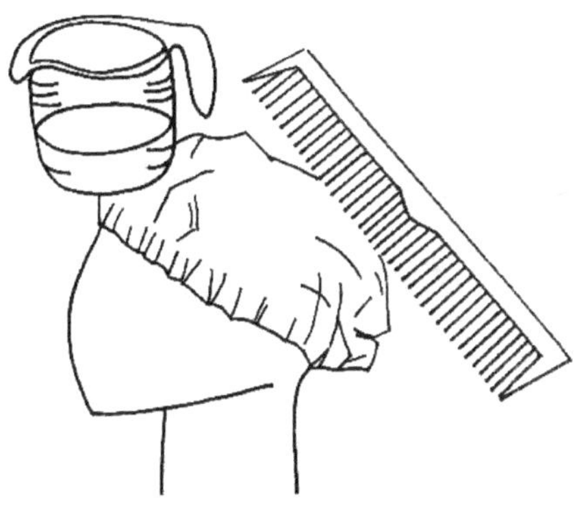

Chapter Nine *What About Your Home* must be completed <u>before</u> you wash the oil or Dimethicone out of your hair.

It can be simpler than you think to get rid of head lice and it costs nearly nothing to do it. First, you will need to gather a few things: a fine-tooth or straight comb, a shower cap, and a suffocant such as Dimethicone or oil, which kill the head lice.

NOTE: *If you have small children, do NOT let them wear the shower cap unsupervised due to the risk of suffocation. Do NOT let them fall asleep or go to bed with a plastic shower cap on.*

Find a place in your house that is well lit (you can never have too much light) and is easy to sweep or vacuum. Depending on the severity of the case, you may find you are sweeping or vacuuming the floor several times throughout the treatment.

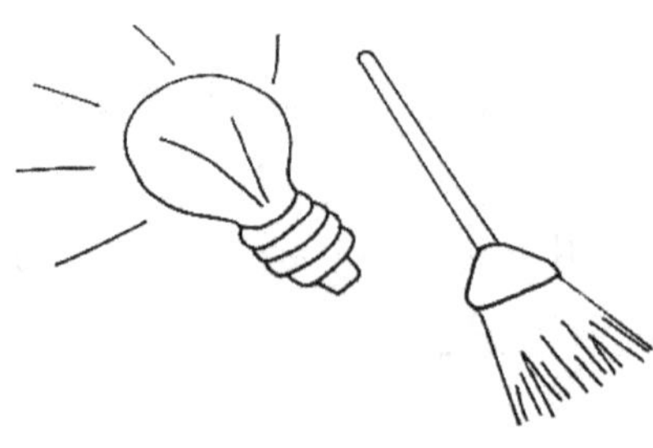

My choice of suffocant is Dimethicone but it's not always easy to find. Also, a very small percentage of people have an adverse/allergic reaction to Dimethicone. If you feel that might be the case, use one of these oils instead: olive oil, coconut oil or vegetable oil. All of these oils will suffocate the bugs completely. This system works because it is based on the lifespan of the head lice bug.

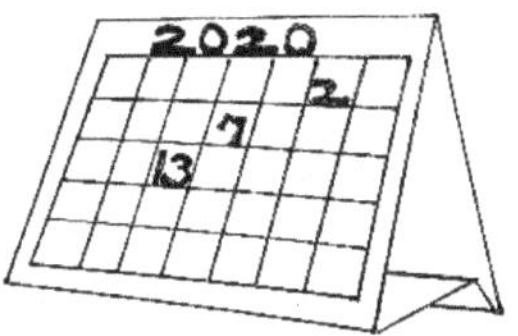

You will be treating yourself only three times: *Day One, Day Five* and *Day Eleven.* All three days are extremely important. You can't miss one of these treatments. Mark them on your calendar.

Day One will kill all the bugs on your head by suffocating them with the oil. If you do a comb out with a lice comb, there is a chance an egg may get left behind. That egg will hatch up to Day ten.

You will be treating yourself two more times with oil or Dimethicone on Day Five and Day Eleven to kill the new hatched eggs. Be assured they will all be hatched and killed on Day Eleven during your final treatment.

.

***

Chapter Seven

The Procedure Step by Step

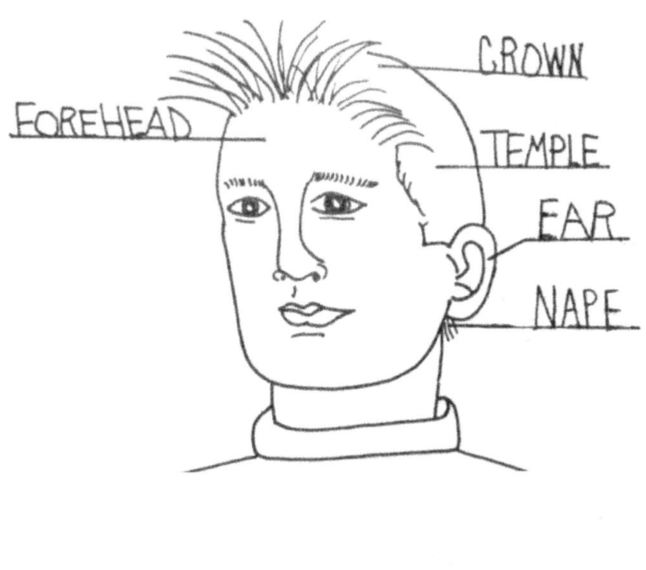

(7a)

Let's Get Started!

Illustration 7a is a simple sketch of the parts of the head I will be referring to in my instructions: FOREHEAD, CROWN, TEMPLE, EAR, and NAPE (or neckline or base) of the neck.

 I've divided the treatment of head lice into three steps: Step 1 and Step 2 are in this Chapter and Step 3 is in Chapter Eight.

If you have a light case of head lice (not severe) and choose not to do a comb out, skip this Chapter (Chapter 7) which covers Steps 1 and 2, and go straight to Chapter Eight which is Step 3.

Speaking from experience, I've gotten head lice several times and have never given myself a comb out.

If you aren't doing your own comb out, make sure the person doing the comb-out is covered with a good fitting shower cap, and that the area bordering the shower cap is outlined with Dimethicone or oil.

Step One

a. ***Mark Day One, Day Five and Day Eleven on your calendar.***

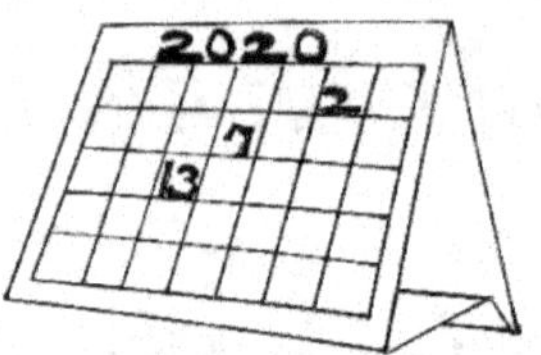

Begin by counting five days after your first treatment. For example, if your first treatment is March 2, Day Five is March 7 and Day Eleven is March 13.

b. *Wash and comb your hair with a <u>straight comb</u>. Diagram 7b.*

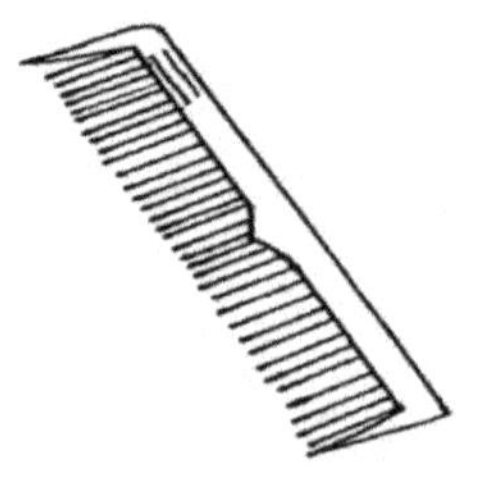

(7b)

c. *Dampen your hair with 1/3 conditioner mixed with 2/3 water (or ½ conditioner with ½ water if you want a stronger mixture.) Mix this in a spray bottle. You will be applying this periodically throughout the procedure, using as needed.*

If you can't get the comb through your hair at all or without a lot of pulling and tugging (and pain), and if your comb has a lot of glue-like residue on it, then you have an <u>extreme case</u> of head lice. Please go to Chapter Twelve where I cover what to do for extreme cases of head lice.

d. Gather the following materials for use in the next steps:

- *a Terminator Nit Free lice comb*
- *paper towels - I prefer using white paper towels as it is easier to see the bugs*
- *zip lock plastic bags (pint size or larger)*
- *a few hair clips*
- *conditioner mix*

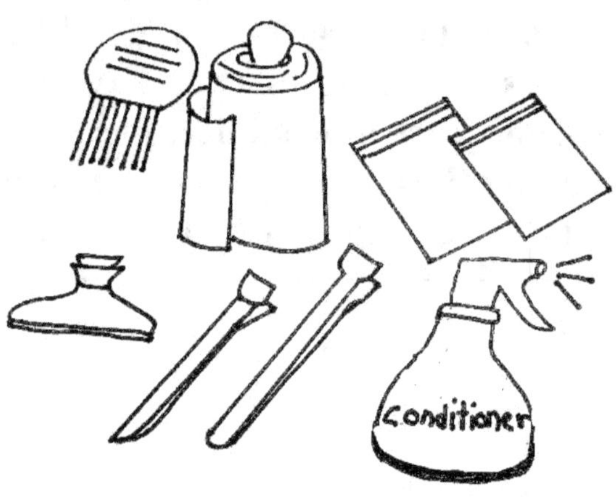

If you want to find every egg, you may want
to include a magnifying glass.

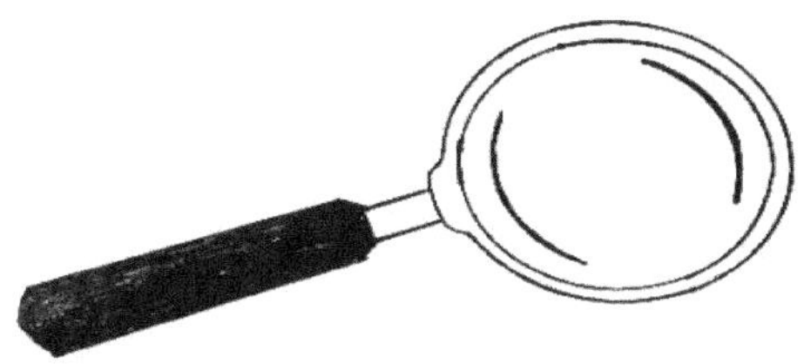

Step 2

The Comb Out

A. *Using a <u>straight comb</u> thoroughly comb your
hair with your conditioner/water mix until it
is damp. Comb from front to back. Start at
your forehead and comb towards the back of
your head as in diagram 7c.*

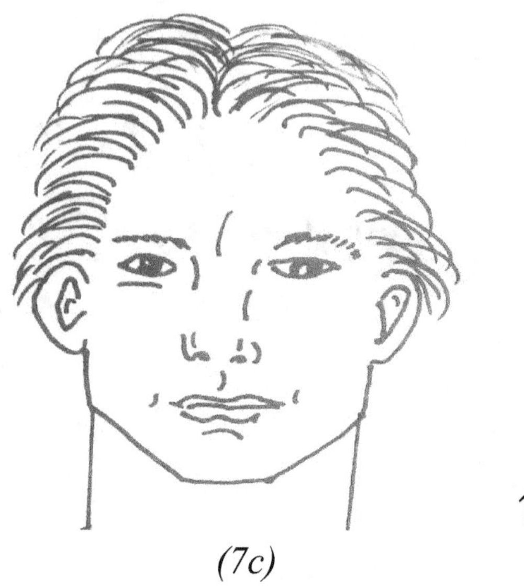

(7c)

B. Now you will use the lice comb.

A good rule to follow is to comb from your scalp, setting the <u>lice comb</u> on the scalp while pulling the comb all the way through the hair.

Begin with the left ear. See diagram 7d.

On the left side of your head, take your <u>lice comb</u> and begin combing around your left ear, hitting all areas in diagram 7d. Start *with upward strokes, pulling out all bugs, eggs and glue.*

The area <u>behind</u> the ear is a favorite lice zone due to the moisture and warmth it provides, so expect to find more nits and bugs there.

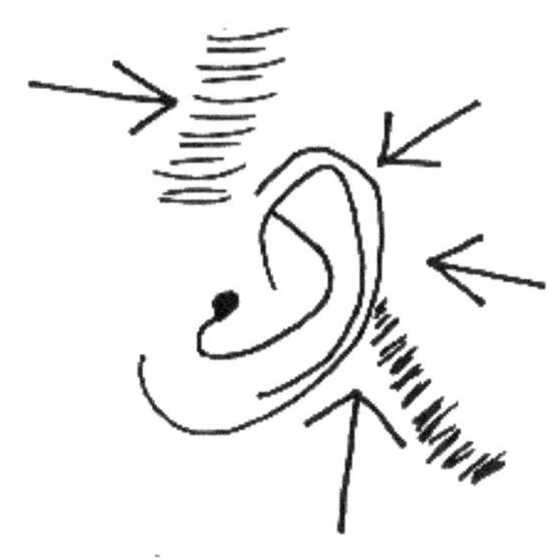

(7d) Left Ear

Wipe any bugs and eggs from the comb on a dry paper towel then place the paper towel in a plastic bag and seal it shut after each swipe.

When you've finished combing with upward strokes, begin combing the same region with downward strokes, (pointing the hair towards the floor and combing downward). When you've completed the downward strokes, repeat the same region with sideways strokes. The reason for this is that eggs are laid on the hair strand in various positions, so combing in all directions guarantees you will get all the eggs.

Repeat this procedure over and over until the comb comes out clean. Give ten more swipes to complete this step.

Nits on hair strands

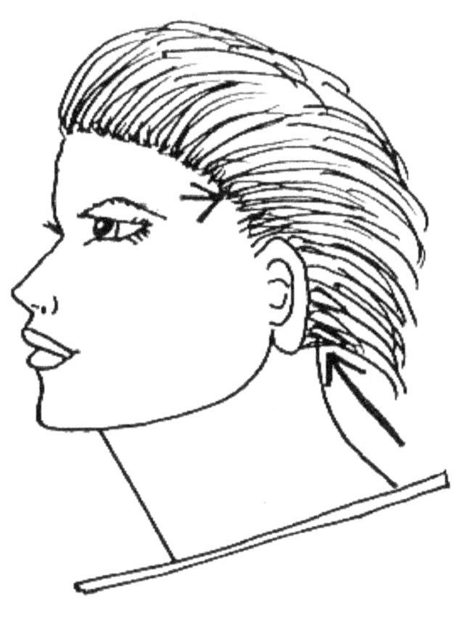

(7e)

C. *Next, move down to the section below the ear,
following the neckline, combing upwards,
downwards and sideways (as stated in Step 2,
B.)*

D. *When the area below your ear is completely
combed out, move up and thoroughly comb
the left temple area and left forehead area
(see illustration 7e) combing upwards,
downwards and sideways, until the whole left*

*side of your head is completely combed clean,
(as stated in Step 2, B.).*

E. *When that area is complete, move to the
forehead region of your head. You want to
comb out your entire forehead area, moving
the comb towards the crown, lifting out bugs
and eggs.*

F. *Begin on the left side of your forehead. Using
your lice comb, start at your forehead
hairline, as in diagram 7f, and placing the
<u>lice comb</u> on the scalp, begin pulling it
through your hair, moving it towards your
crown.*

*Remember to comb the individual areas in all
directions, beginning with upward strokes,
then downward strokes* (pointing the hair
towards the floor and combing downward)
then sideways strokes, until the comb comes

out clean. Give ten extra swipes to complete the step.

G. *Repeat the procedure in the right forehead region.*

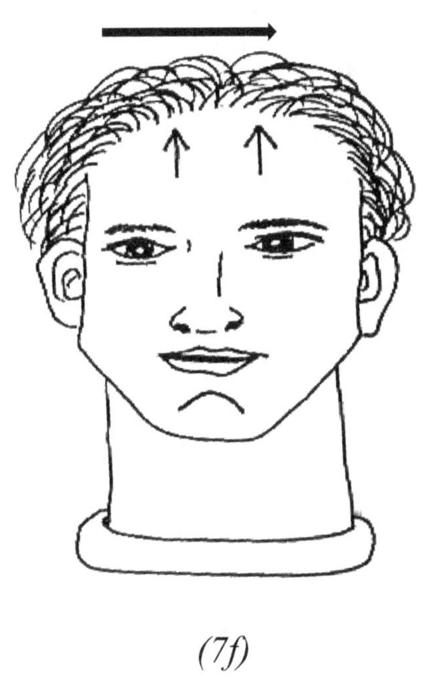

(7f)

H. *Once the forehead area is finished, move to the right side of your head, and comb around the ear, as you did in step B. Complete steps*

C and D, ending with ten extra swipes for good measure.

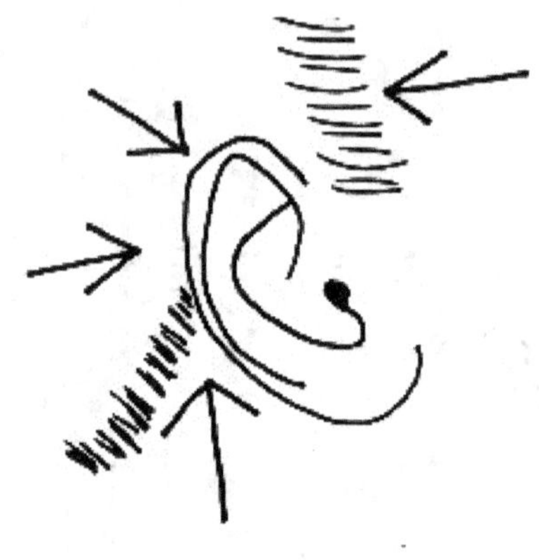

(7g)

Right Ear

I. *When the right ear area is complete, go to the* **right** *side of your head and using your* <u>straight comb</u> *(see diagram 7b), comb* <u>all</u> *your hair to the* **left** *side of your head, as diagram 7h shows. Use your conditioner mix as needed to keep the hair moist.*

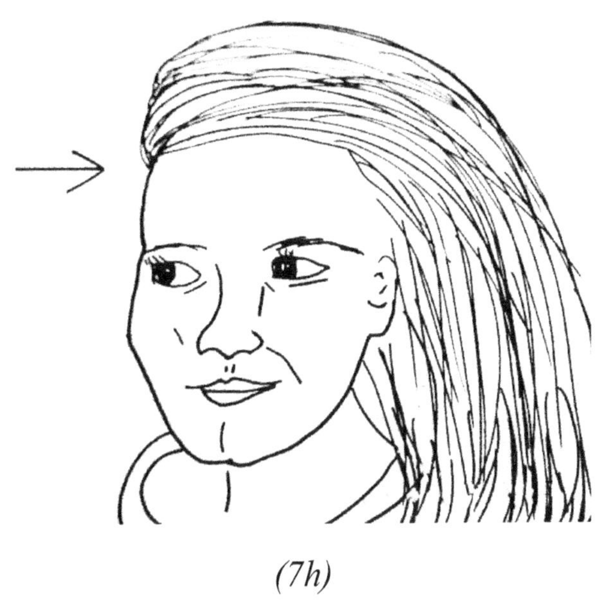

(7h)

J. *Now, using your <u>lice comb</u>, start with a one-inch section at the nape of your neck on the right side, and pull the comb all the way through the hair towards the left side of your head, removing eggs and bugs. Do this every direction until your lice comb comes out clean.*

K. *Next, continuing with the <u>lice comb</u>, move up the nape of the neck an inch, and comb another one-inch section, combing through it thoroughly. Then, move up another inch and* comb through that area thoroughly. Keep combing thoroughly, moving up an inch at a time unto you reach the forehead hair line. This removes lice and eggs from the nape of the neck and the hair around the ears and forehead. End the procedure with ten extra swipes for good measure.

L. Repeat this procedure on the left side of your head. See diagram 7i.

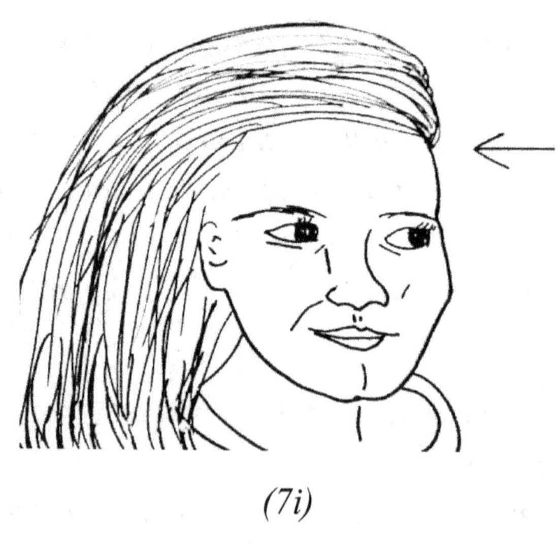

(7i)

M. Next, to remove lice and nits in the middle of
your head, part the hair down the middle
from front to back. See diagram 7j.

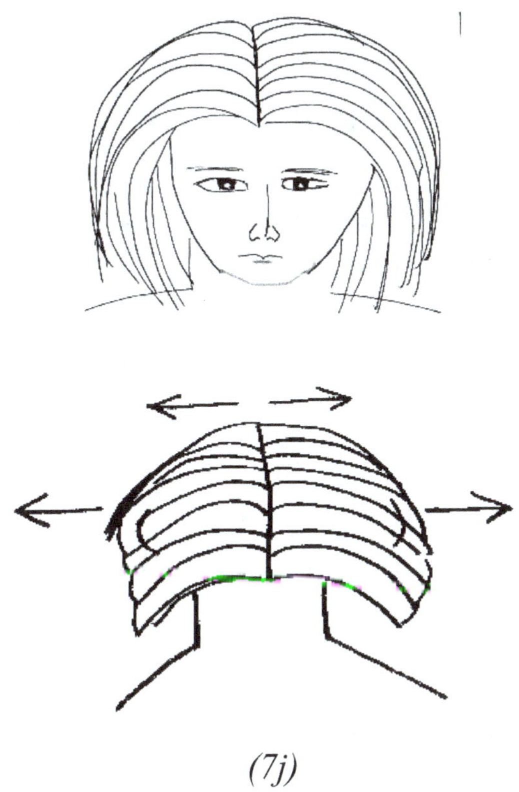

(7j)

N. *Clip the **right** side with hair clips, so it stays out of your way, as you will be combing the **left** side first.*

   *Start at the nape of the neck, and using your <u>lice comb</u>, comb **from the part in the middle** of your head to the left side of the head, pulling the hair all the way through the comb, grabbing bugs and eggs.*

   Continue until no more eggs or bugs are found.

O. *Continue on up the part in sections, combing out eggs and bugs, until you reach the front forehead hair line.*

P. *Once that is completed, clip the hair on the left side of the head, and start on the right side, following steps N-and O.*

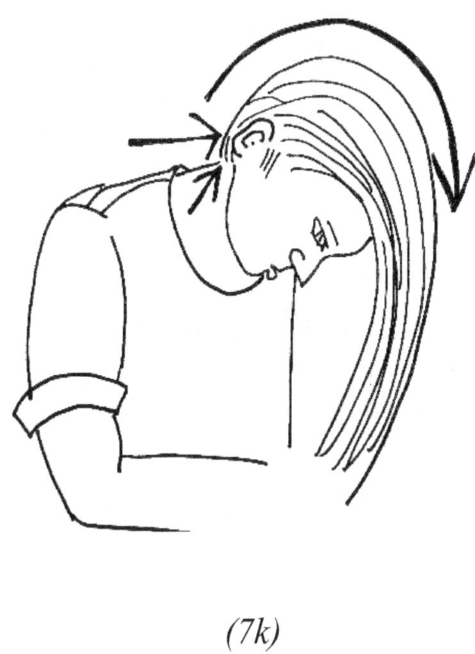

(7k)

*Q. When that is completed, you will need to get rid of the eggs and nits along your <u>neckline</u>. Using a <u>straight comb</u>, **comb your hair over your head.** This may be difficult if you have long hair, but it is necessary as the neckline is a favorite place for head lice to breed due to the warmth it provides for them.*

R. Next, use your <u>lice comb</u>, and starting from the left side of the nape of the neck, comb up, *bringing the comb all the way through the hair. It may take many swipes to get all the eggs and bugs, as lice prefer the neckline due to the moisture and heat the hair provides.*

When your comb comes out clean, move an inch to the right, pulling eggs and bugs out with your lice comb. Keep inching over until the whole neckline is clean.

Then give it ten extra swipes for good measure.

Make sure you don't miss any of the hairs around your hair line. Every strand of hair, even the tiny loose hairs in the front, ear area and back of your head, can have lice eggs. Use your fingernails if the eggs seem to slip through the comb.

That completes Steps 1 and 2

and your comb out.

***

Chapter Eight

Step Three

"Suffocant"

Do Step Three on days 1, 5, and 11.

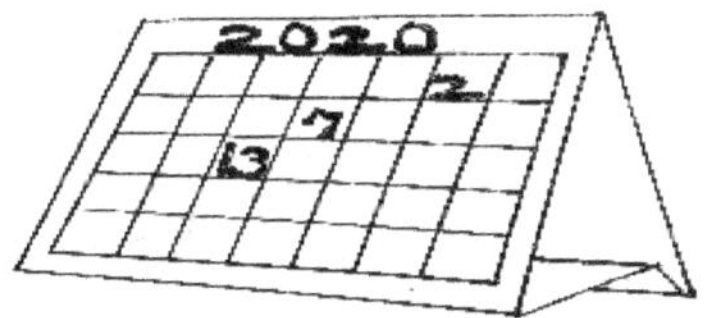

Begin by marking your calendar, counting five days after your first treatment. For example, if your first treatment is March 2, Day Five is March 7 and Day Eleven is March 13.

You may want to protect your clothes by placing an apron, towel or garbage bag over you.

For this Step, you will start with clean, combed and slightly damp hair. **For people with <u>kinky, coily or natural hair</u> who don't or can't comb through their hair, start with clean and slightly damp hair.**

(If you used a brush on your hair before you combed it, place it in your freezer overnight to kill any eggs or bugs that may be on it).

1. If your hair is a little dry, dampen it. Just damp…. not dripping wet

2. You will need two or more ounces of Dimethicone or ¼ cup of oil of your choice (olive, melted coconut, vegetable, almond).

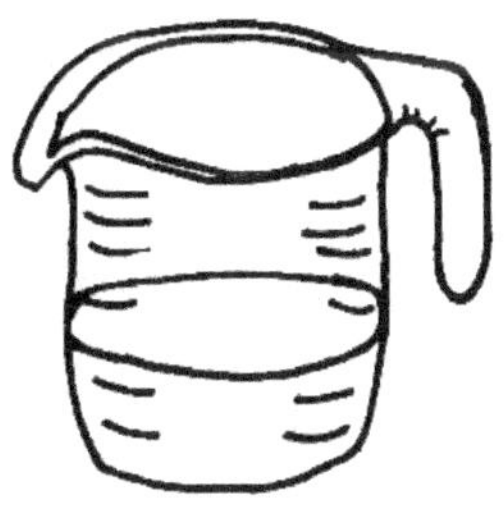

3. Starting at the crown of your head, pour a few tablespoons of Dimethicone or an oil of your choice onto your hair and rub it in.

4. Next, pour a few tablespoons in the hair around each ear and rub thoroughly into that area.

5. Then, pour a few tablespoons into the nape of the neck and rub in that area thoroughly.

6. Use your fingers to remove the rest of the oil or Dimethicone from the container (or get more if you have used it all) and pour that over your head randomly, rubbing it in thoroughly onto your entire scalp and hair.

Use as much oil as you need to *fully saturate* the hair and scalp. It is better to have too much than too little.

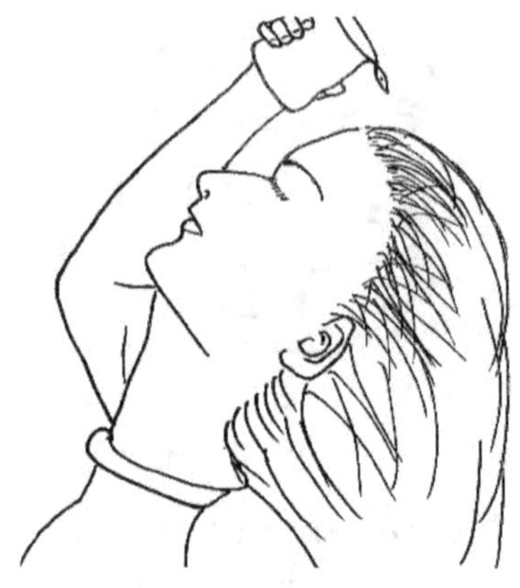

7. Next, use your <u>straight comb</u> (diagram 7b) and *thoroughly* comb the oil or Dimethicone into your hair, until your ENTIRE scalp and EVERY strand of hair is thoroughly covered in the Dimethicone or oil.

> **For people with <u>kinky, coily or natural hair</u> who don't or can't brush or comb through their hair, use your fingers to work the oil through your hair and scalp. Use as much oil as you need, covering every hair strand and your entire scalp. See Chapter Five for more information.**

Take your time.

Begin with the thick tines on your comb, then switch to the fine tines to thoroughly comb all the oil into your hair and scalp.

8. Use more oil or Dimethicone if your hair is extra-long or thick. With thick hair, make sure the back of the head is thoroughly covered. You may have to section the hair off to make sure nothing is left un-oiled. Use less oil or Dimethicone for short or fine hair. If you think you may need more, add more. It doesn't hurt if too much oil or Dimethicone is added to the hair.

9. When the oil is all combed in and your hair looks completely shiny and greasy clear down to the scalp, cover your head with a shower cap and leave it in your hair NO LESS than **one hour** for Dimethicone and **eight hours** for the oils. (I've fallen asleep with Dimethicone in my hair and washed it out the next morning with no problems).

<u>DIMETHICONE</u>
1-hour

<u>OIL</u>
8-hours

NOTE: *If you have <u>small children</u>, do NOT let them wear the shower cap unsupervised due to the risk of suffocation. Do NOT let them fall asleep or go to bed with a plastic shower cap on!*

10. Once the cap is on your head—change your clothes! There is a good chance there are bugs on your clothes. Place your clothes in the dryer right away, or in a safe place where they won't touch anything, such as a sealed plastic bag.

11. Next, follow the instructions in Chapter 9 *What About My Home*, and after your house is lice-safe, wash out your hair per these instructions:

*Remember, you have OIL (or Dimethicone) in your hair so **DO NOT apply water**—yet.*

How to Wash Out Your Hair

a. First, apply a good measure of DISH SOAP into your hair and work it in thoroughly. Use a dish soap that cuts grease well, like Blue Dawn dish soap. If you are concerned that dish soap may be too harsh on your children, use their favorite shampoo.

b. AFTER the dish soap is amply applied and worked through your hair, rinse it out with water. You can shampoo your hair following this if you want to. The house is safe. Your hair is safe for now. Relax.

12. Repeat Chapter 8 in **FIVE DAYS**.

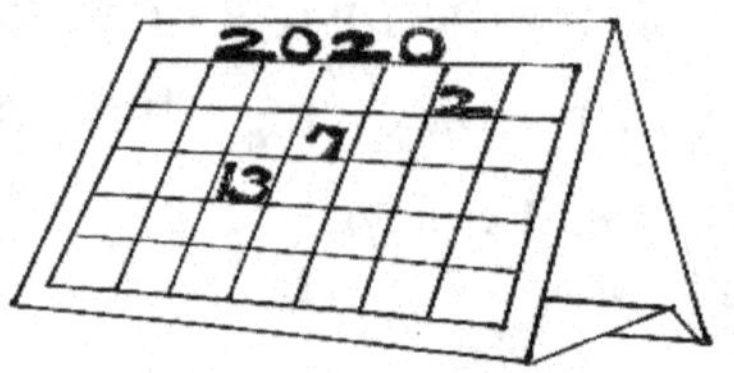

Begin by counting five days after your first treatment. For example, if your first treatment is March 2, Day Five is March 7 and Day Eleven is March 13.

13. Repeat Chapter 8 in **SIX DAYS** (this is the 11th day).

Why is the 11th day so very important?

Because every egg will be hatched by this day, and the oil or Dimethicone will suffocate them before they have a chance to mature and lay more eggs.

You are now officially "Lice Free!"

***

Chapter Nine

What About Your Home?

All you need is a **clothes dryer, freezer, lint roller** and **vacuum cleaner**.

That's it!

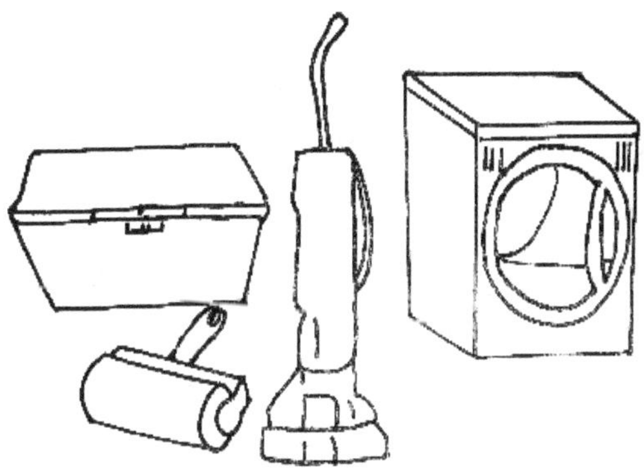

These next steps must be done your *first day* <u>before</u> you wash the oil out of your hair. I recommend you also repeat these steps on Days Five and Eleven.

You don't need to tear your house apart but be thorough. Remember, head lice are dead in 48 hours once they are off a host (us).

You can technically close up entire rooms in your house for 48 hours and not do a thing to them, and every bug will be dead.

What about the eggs? Eggs need a warm, moist environment to hatch. Upon hatching, they must IMMEDIATELY eat (your blood is their food supply). If these 3 things aren't available to them (warmth, moisture, blood) they cannot survive upon hatching. You need to decide if your rooms are at risk of lice eggs hatching in them.

Steps to a Bug Free Home

1. Every floor needs to be vacuumed or swept.

2. All furniture you've sat or laid on must be lint rolled or vacuumed.

3. The Last 48 hours of <u>clothes</u> need to be in the dryer for 30 min on your HOTTEST setting (125° F) or placed in your freezer or outdoors in 25° F or less weather overnight.

4. All <u>bedding</u> needs to be in the dryer for 30 minutes on hottest setting (125° F or hotter) or placed in your freezer or outdoors in 25° F or colder, overnight. This includes <u>pillows and stuffed animals</u> your children slept with. Anything they haven't touched in the last 48 hours is safe from bugs.

For <u>pillows or stuffed animals</u> that cannot go in the driver or freezer, thoroughly lint roll them or place them in a plastic bag for 12 days.

5. <u>Combs, brushes and hair accessories</u> need to be placed in the freezer overnight.

6. Anything that has been placed on the head, such as <u>scarves, helmets, caps, hats</u>, etc. need to be placed in the dyer, freezer, dishwasher, or lint rolled thoroughly before placing back

on the head, or place them in a plastic bag for 12 days.

Don't Forget the Car!

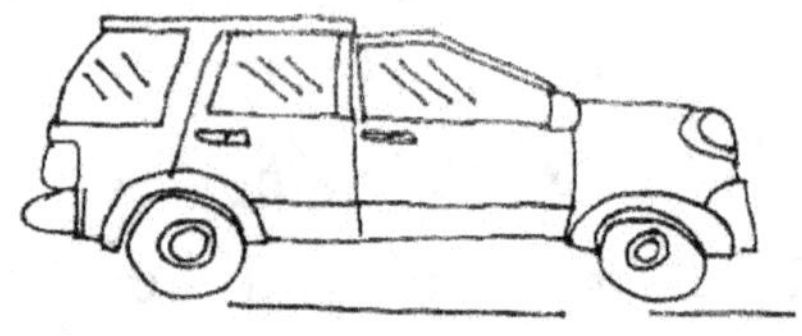

NOTE: Lice will freeze to death in 25°F or lower temperatures. If your car will be outside in this temperature, it is safe. You won't need to vacuum, or lint roll it. If the temperatures are above freezing, vacuum and lint roll your interior, focusing on the head rests and car seats.

***

Chapter Ten

How to Prevent Future Head Lice Infestations.

How do I protect myself and my family from getting head lice again?

There is no guarantee you won't get head lice again, but there are excellent ways to protect yourself against it.

1. Brush your hair daily. *Be very thorough.* Brush from the scalp all the way down to the ends of your hair, using a hairbrush with *a lot* of bristles. Think *Boar Bristle* hairbrush. The bristles need to be firm enough to penetrate your scalp. If you have thick hair, you need medium to firm hair bristles. It is conceivable that you may have contacted head lice, and you need a hairbrush that can lift them out of your hair.

When you're done brushing, clean the hair out of the brush, flush it, or take it outside to the garbage can, then stick the brush in the freezer overnight. Repeat next day.

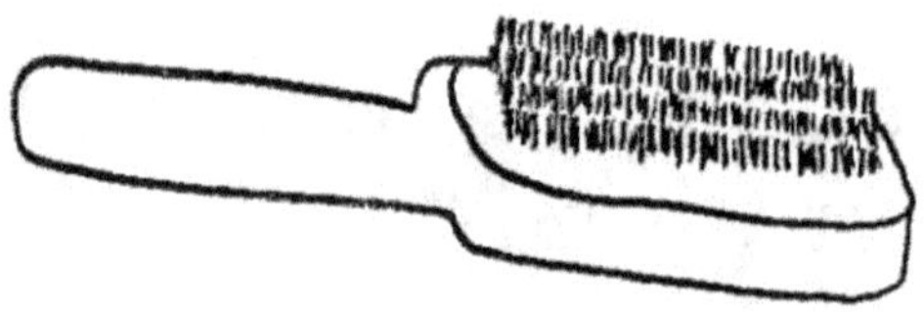

2. Don't share brushes. Each family member should have their own hairbrush.

3. Check yourself and your family *regularly* with a good head lice comb. I recommend that Terminator Nit Free Head Lice comb.

It can be a weekly or bi-weekly head check. You decide what works best for you and your family. Be sure to check the most vulnerable places: around the ears, neck and crown of head. It should take you less than a minute or two.

4. Use hair products such as mousse, gels, leave-on conditioners, hair sprays, styling creams, etc. Head lice thrive in clean hair— although they are found in dirty hair, also. Using hair products is a good deterrent but not a fail-safe remedy.

5. Use hair dryers, straighteners, curling irons, etc. Lice hate the heat.

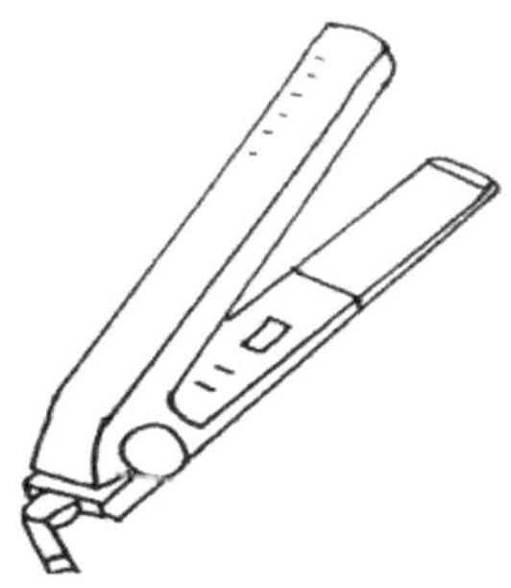

6. Keep long hair tied back in braids or in buns. Remember, lice swing from hair strand to hair strand. If your hair is tight to your head, they have a difficult time moving around. Braids and buns are an excellent protection.

7. Wear hats! Baseball caps, scarves, cowboy hats, etc. Make it difficult for lice to swing onto your hair.

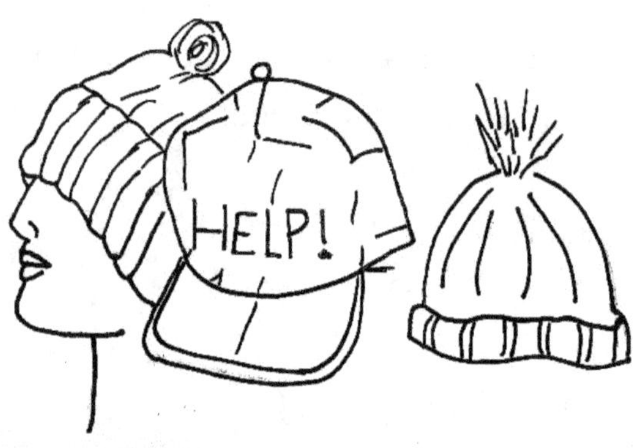

8. Never go to bed with wet hair. Head lice need a warm, moist environment to thrive. Don't provide that for them.

9. Essential Oils! Tea tree oil, lavender oil, rosemary oil…. Lice HATE these! I spray my hair with rosemary/lavender oil. It's easy to prepare and a little goes a LONG way! Spray whenever you feel you may be at risk for getting head lice. Note: these don't kill head lice, but they are a deterrent. I don't

guarantee you won't get head lice from using these, but the odds of you getting them are decreased dramatically. I cover more about this in Chapter Eleven.

10. Check your children and yourself for head lice after sleepovers, camp outs, or when you or they have been with friends that may be at risk.

***

Chapter Eleven

Essential Oils

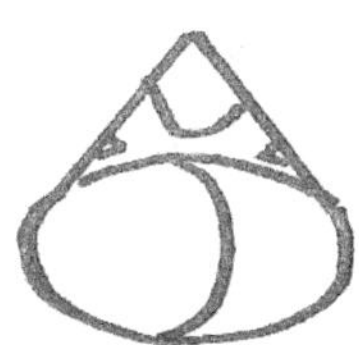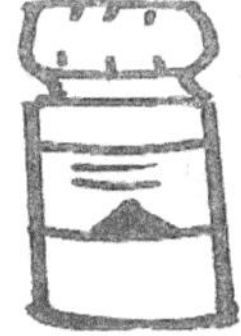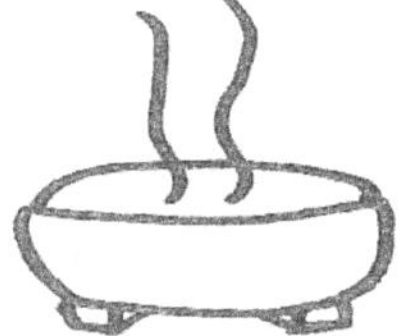

What are Essential Oils? An essential oil is a natural oil derived from the plant from which it was extracted, such as oil of rosemary. The oil contains the "essence" of the plant's fragrance.

Tea Tree Oil is probably the most popular essential oil used in treating head lice. It has natural insecticide properties that repel head lice. Most of my clients with head lice have used tea tree oil and I still find head lice on them. Therefore, I recommend it as a preventive measure, not as an oil that will kill them.

I've heard remarkable stories from my clients who used Tea Tree as a preventive measure.

If you are someone who works around head lice on a daily basis, such as in a day care, I highly recommend using tea tree oil daily. If you cannot tolerate its unique fragrance, there are other essentials oils you can use. My favorite is a combination of rosemary and lavender oil.

Rosemary/Lavender Oil. I make up my own using 1/4th cup of distilled water and 10 drops of Rosemary and 10 drops of lavender. Shake before using and keep it in a cool place. I spray my hair before going out or seeing clients. I have many clients who spray their children daily before sending them off to school or camp.

Some people like adding an essential oil to their treatment. Be sure it is safe for your hair, scalp and skin before using.

There is more information about essential oils and head lice online.

***

Chapter Twelve

Severe Cases of Head Lice

In my eight years of treating head lice I have come across only five families who had, what I would call, a severe case of head lice. If you are wondering if you have an extreme case, try this test.

Take a fine-tooth comb and begin combing around your ears. If you can't get the comb through your hair at all or without a lot of pulling and tugging (and pain), and if your comb has a lot of glue-like residue on it, then you have an extreme case of head lice.

What happens in severe cases like this is the lice lay many eggs on a single strand of hair. Times that with a thousand(s) strands of hair and you literally have layers of eggs and glue in your hair.

To add insult to injury, it is not unusual to find bugs between the layers of glue and eggs.

It can be very laborious and painful to get rid of all the eggs, bugs and glue; but with persistence you will end up with a clean, lice-free scalp.

The key? Don't give up!

To begin, buy a Terminator Nit Free comb.

Next, read Chapter Seven, especially Steps 1 and 2, and follow the instructions in Step One.

Keep in mind, a lot varies with the thickness of the hair. The thicker the hair, the longer it takes to remove the eggs.

If you can, get someone to help you. Provide a snug shower cap and an apron or plastic covering to protect their hair and clothes.

Choose a location in the house that is well lit and where it is easy to sweep up the lice that may land on the floor.

COMBING PROCESS:

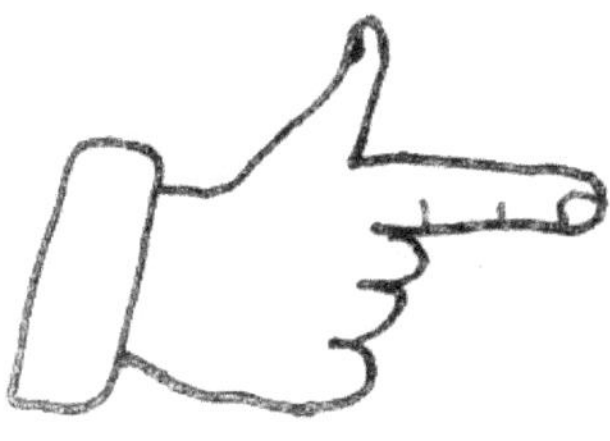

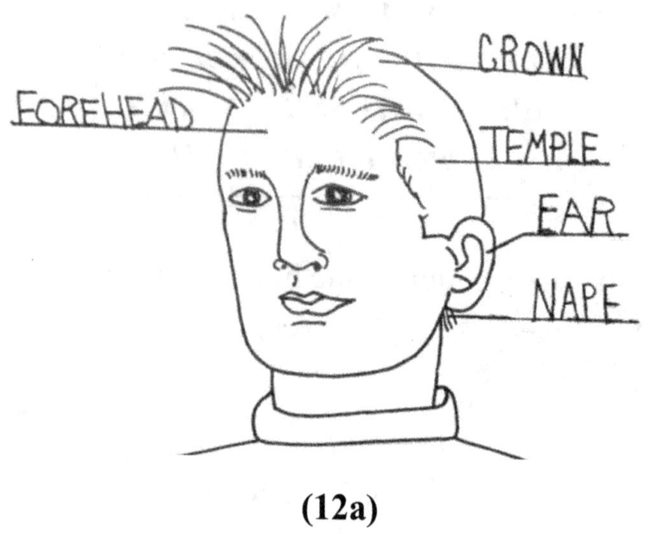

(12a)

This is a simple sketch of the parts of the head I will be referring to in my instructions: FOREHEAD, CROWN, TEMPLE, EAR, and NAPE of neck (or NECKLINE).

It's important to section small amounts of hair and clean out the lice bugs and eggs in that area thoroughly.

Step A: The Forehead Line

1. Dampen the hair with the conditioner/water mix as explained in Chapter 7.

2. Comb all the hair straight back with your straight comb. (Diagram 7b) Divide your hair in 2-inch segments along your forehead. (See diagram 12b).

3. Starting at the left (#1 in the diagram), begin at the forehead and move two inches down only. Use your clips to clip back any hair that may fall outside the 2x2 area in section 1.

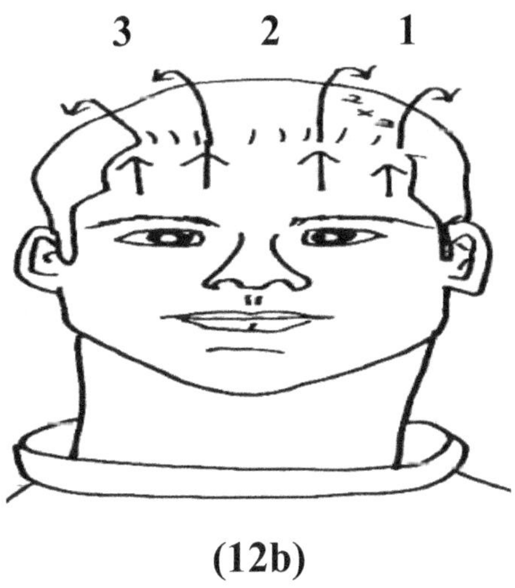

(12b)

4. You will comb out head lice and eggs in this 2x2 area with your <u>head lice comb,</u> combing in all directions (up, down, and sideways) to assure all bugs, glue and eggs are cleaned out.

Comb from your scalp, (set the lice comb on the scalp) pulling the comb all the way through the hair, using upward strokes.

When you've finished combing with upward strokes, begin combing the same region with downward strokes, (pointing the hair towards the floor and combing downward). When you've completed the downward strokes, repeat the same region with sideways strokes.

The reason for this is that eggs are laid on the hair strand in various positions, so combing in all directions guarantees you will get all the eggs.

Repeat this procedure over and over until the comb comes out clean. Give ten more swipes for good measure.

5. When done, move down the head *directly beneath the area you just cleaned,* clipping off another 2x2 area to comb. Make sure it is *directly beneath the first area.* Comb that area out like you did the first area in step 4.

Repeat this procedure, moving down the head until you reach the nape of the neck. The neckline often has a lot of eggs, so be thorough when combing this area. The neckline is a very painful area because of the many tiny hairs in that area, but don't give up! You will succeed.

6. When you've completed Section 1, start at Section 2 at the forehead line again, (to the right of the 2x2 area in the diagram) moving to the right, as shown in the picture, and comb as you did the first section, all the way to the nape of the neck.

Then repeat, doing section 3.

 If your forehead is wide, you may have a section 4 or 5.

Complete until the forehead line is done.

____

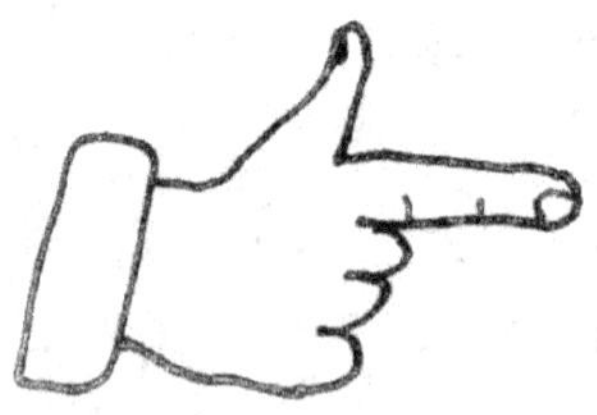

Step B: The Side of the Head

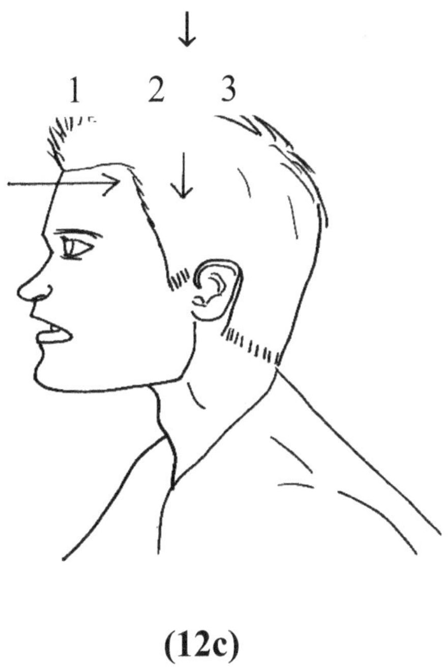

(12c)

Begin at the forehead line where it meets the temple. You'll be moving down the left side of the head, combing out 2x2 segments, just like in the previous step.

Move down the head *directly beneath the*

area you just cleaned, clipping off another 2x2 area to comb. Make sure it is *directly beneath the first area.*

When you reach the ear area, you will possibly find a lot more glue, bugs and eggs. This can be very painful but be persistent.

Comb in all directions, as in Step A, until your comb comes out clean.

When the left side is complete, (finishing clear down to the ear area and left side neckline,) move over to the right side of the head and repeat this step.

Step C: The Forehead and Back of The Head

This next section may seem redundant, but I have found it extremely helpful in severe cases of head lice.

Steps A and B of this chapter had you working vertically to get rid of bugs, glue and eggs. This step is very similar except you will be combing out using *horizontal lines*.
See diagrams 12d and 12e

1. Let's begin with the Forehead again.
Make a horizontal part with your <u>straight</u> <u>comb</u> clear across the forehead line (see the arrow in diagram 12d). Your part with the straight comb will cross the entire scalp. For example, you will make a straight part from the left temple to the right temple, or from the left ear to the right ear. Etc. (See diagram 12d)

Comb out the eggs, bugs and glue in that area. Comb in all directions, as in Step A, until your comb comes out clean.

2. When you're finished with step 1 along the forehead line, clip that hair back, then proceed an inch underneath that area, and

comb out the bugs, eggs and glue thoroughly.

3. When you're finished with step 2, make another horizontal part one inch beneath that line, heading towards the back of your head, (diagram 12e) and comb out thoroughly. Repeat this, inch by inch, until you reach the neckline.

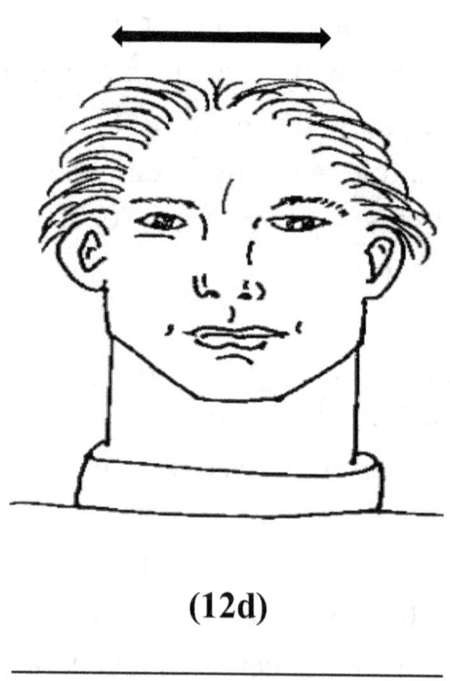

(12d)

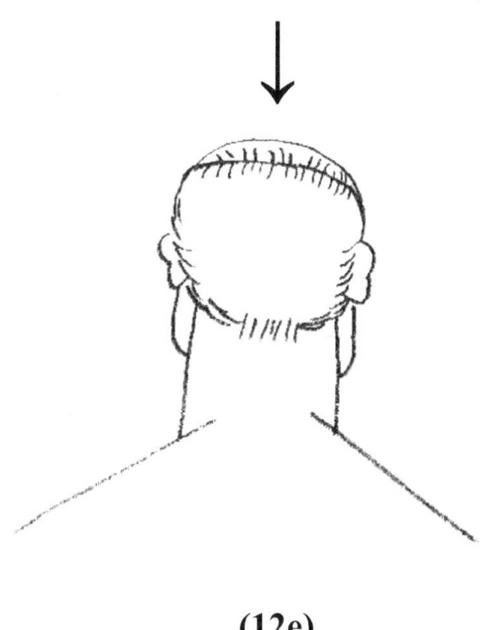

(12e)

Make sure you don't miss any of the hairs around your hair line.

Every strand of hair, even the tiny loose hairs in the front and back of your head, can have eggs.

Double check your hair line!

When you are finished, you will be able to comb through the entire scalp with your <u>straight comb</u> and even your <u>lice comb</u> with ease.

If you have completed these steps, then commend yourself!

No one understands the pain and determination it takes to get rid of a severe case of head lice unless you have been there.

The worst part is over.

Congratulations!

Now Proceed to **Step 3** in Chapter Eight and follow through on Day One, Five and Eleven.

***

If you have any questions, email me at
headlicehelp@yahoo.com or visit my website
www.helpihaveheadlice.com.

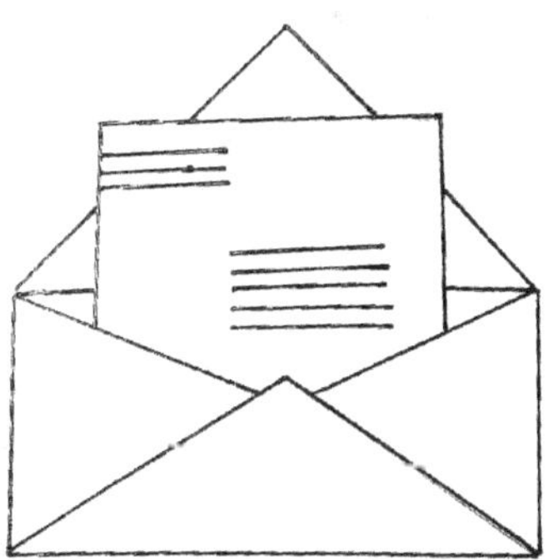

PART II:

A Children's Story

Help!
I Have Head Lice

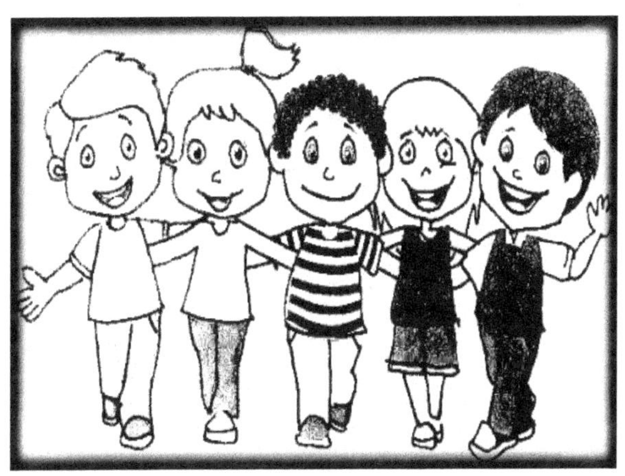

By Bev Gipson

Illustrated by Shannon Hartup

Yikes!

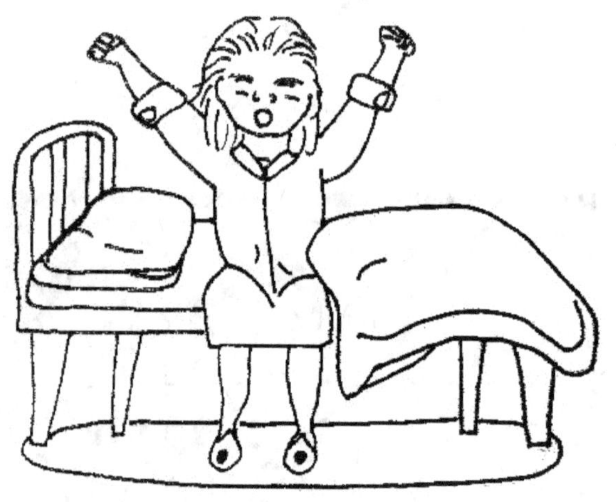

I just now woke up.
I jumped straight out of bed
I'm feeling all itchy
All over my head.

I'm scratching and scratching,
And something's not right
My hair's all a mess
Did I just feel a bite?

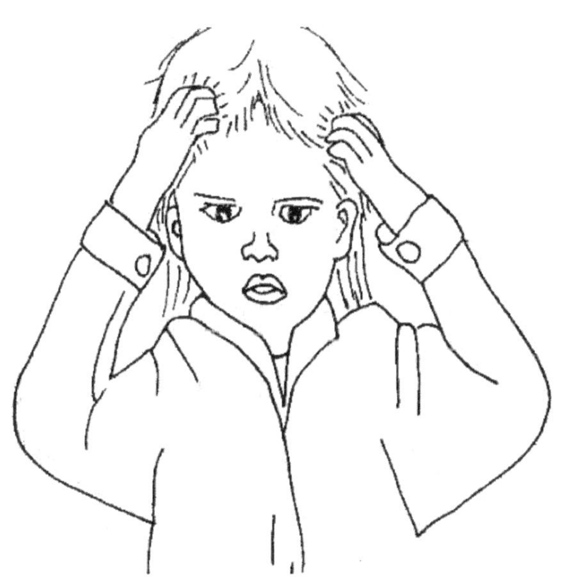

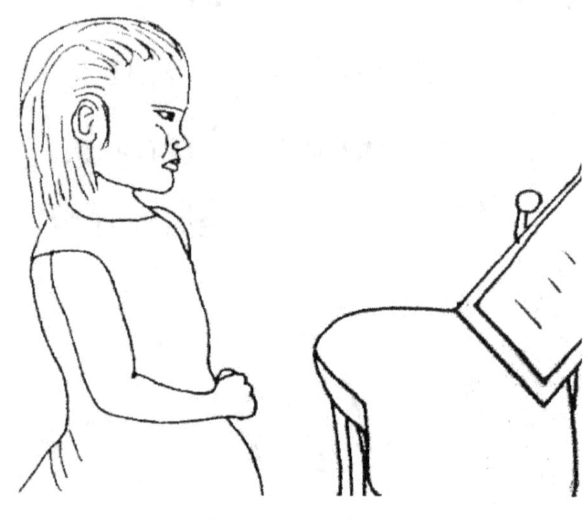

I felt something tickling
And moving my hair
When I looked in the mirror
Nothing was there

.

I ran and told mom
Who started brushing my hair,

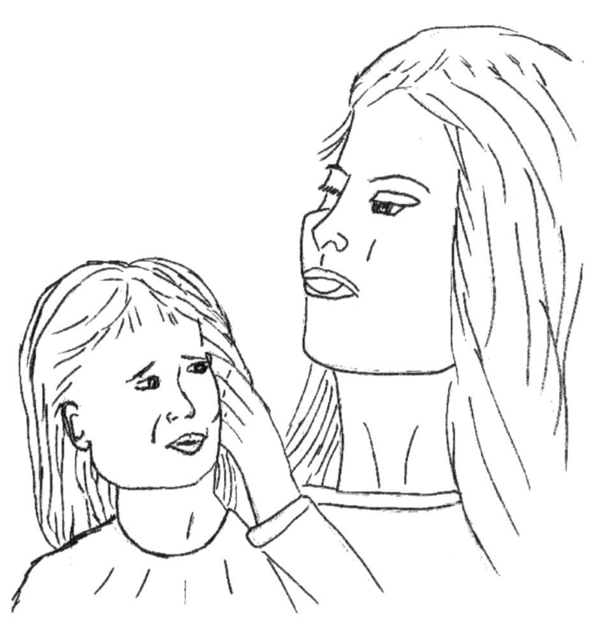

She found a bug here,
And another bug there.

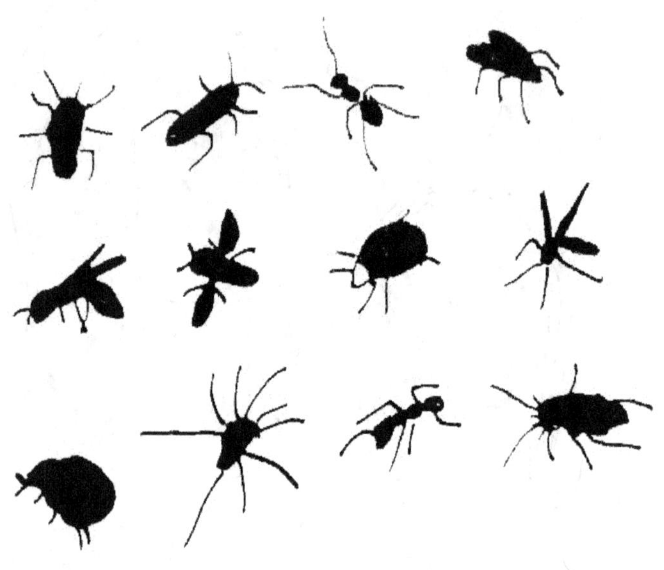

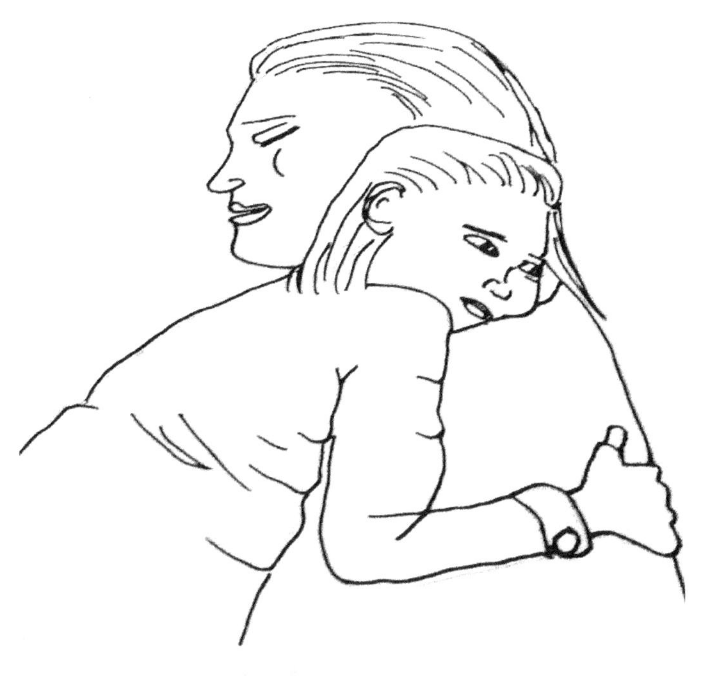

I started to shriek,
I started to cry.
My mom gave me a hug
And I said, "Oh, why?

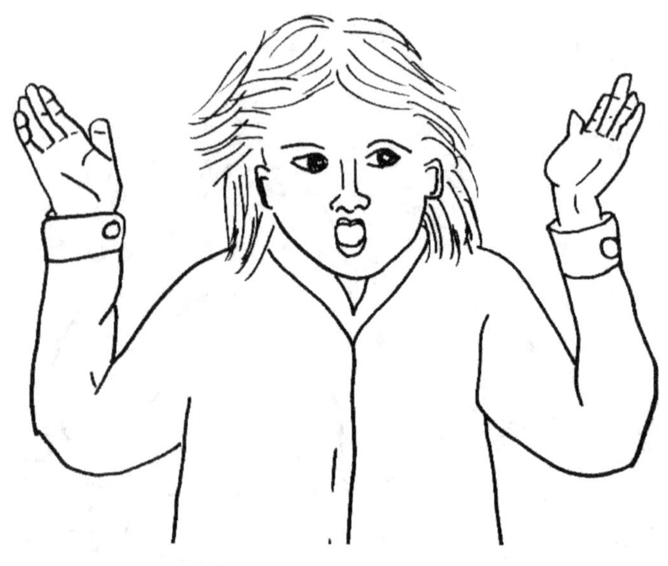

'Why are bugs in my hair?"
"Make those bugs go away!"
"Where did they come from?"
"Are they going to stay?"

Mom knew of those bugs,
"Those pesky head lice!
They won't treat you kindly.
They won't treat you nice!"

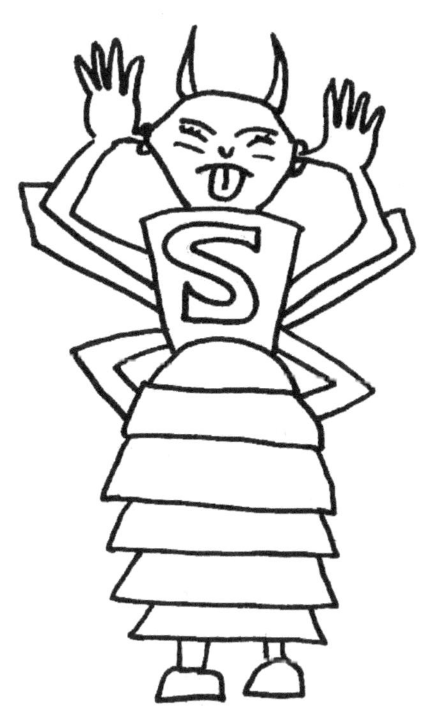

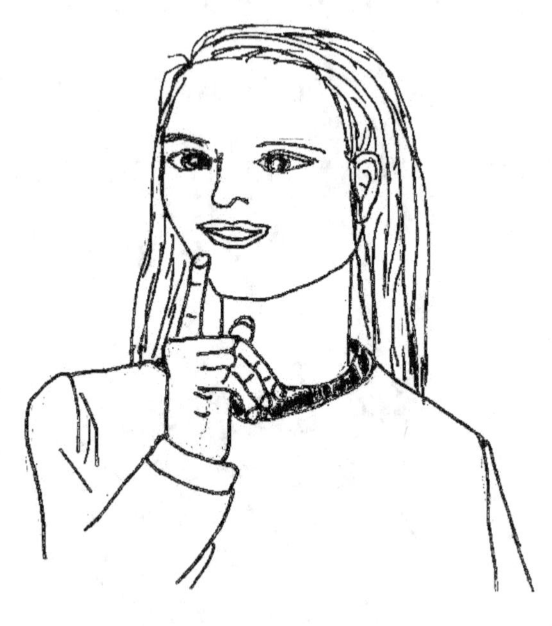

Mom was upset
And I was too
Until she decided
just what we should do.

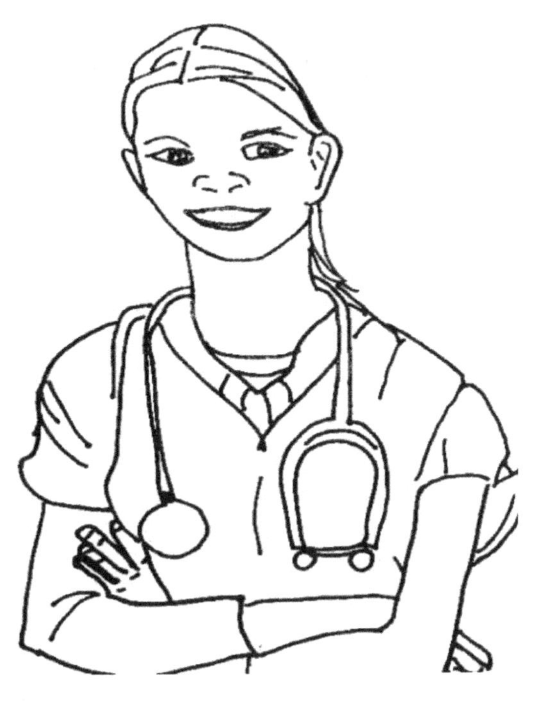

She made a phone call
to a technician,
Who knew how to help
relieve the condition.

An appointment was made
No wait time at all.
I sat by the door
awaiting the call.

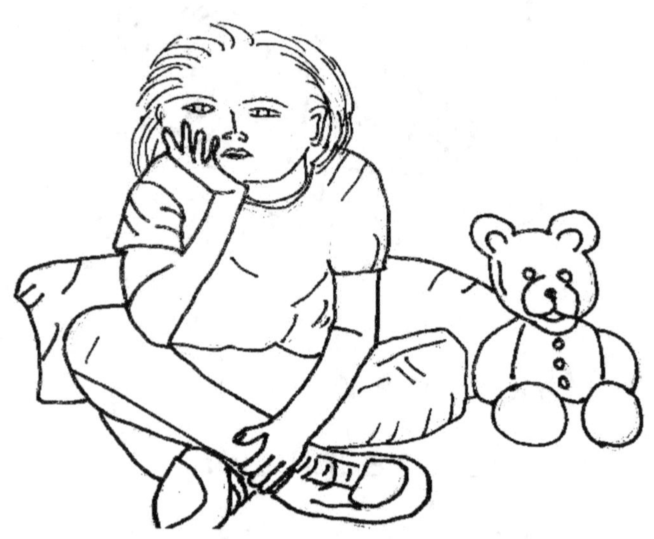

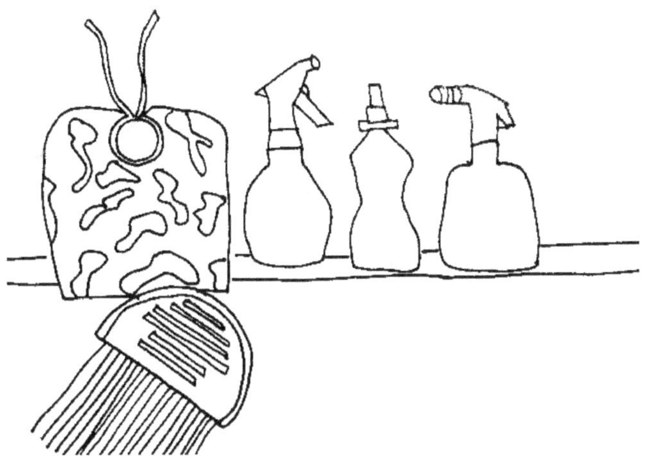

Her basket of bottles
Numbering three
A comb and a cape
She began helping me

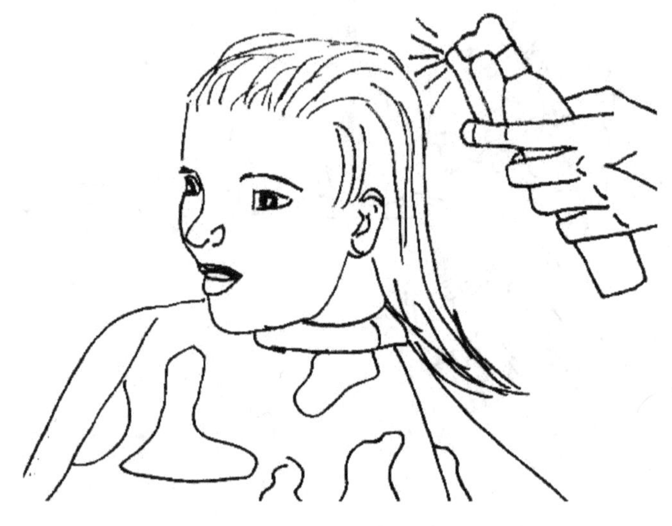

She inspected my head
And combed carefully
And gently applied
Dimethicone to me

Upon my head
She put a cap for a shower
And then let me play
And read for an hour

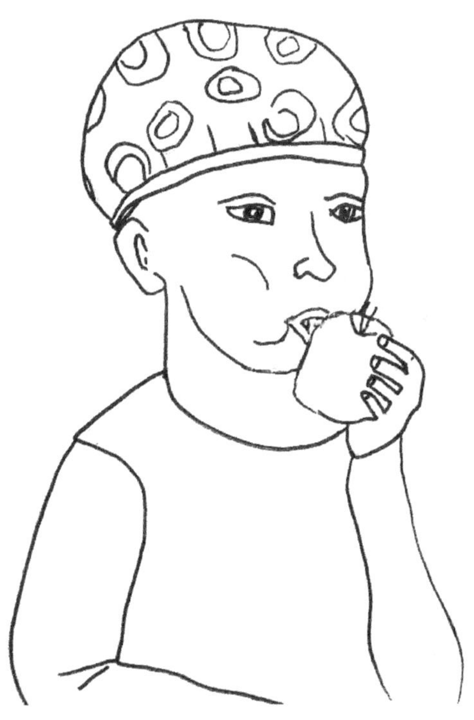

Afterward, my mom
Shampooed me with Dawn
And my, oh, my....
My itch was all gone!

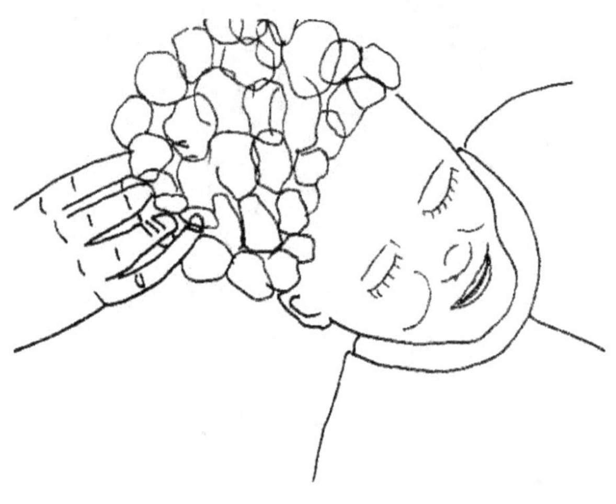

Thank you to all,
I am now bug free.
I can't wait to tell friends and
family!

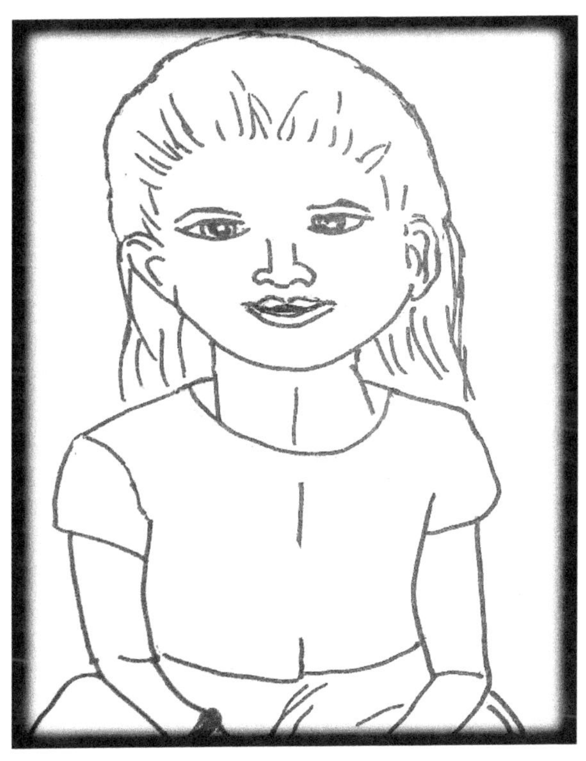

NOTES

NOTES